Sex Positions Coloring Book

Sexy Coloring Book for Adults

JANE SOLOMON

This page intentionally left blank.

ABOUT THE BOOK

This collection of hot couples illustrations for coloring is sure to heat up any night. Get out your crayons and get in a playful mood. Whether it's at a yacht, the beach, the office or at a sexy nightclub these hot men and women are sure to arouse the sensual side in yourself.

CONTENTS

This page intentionally left blank.

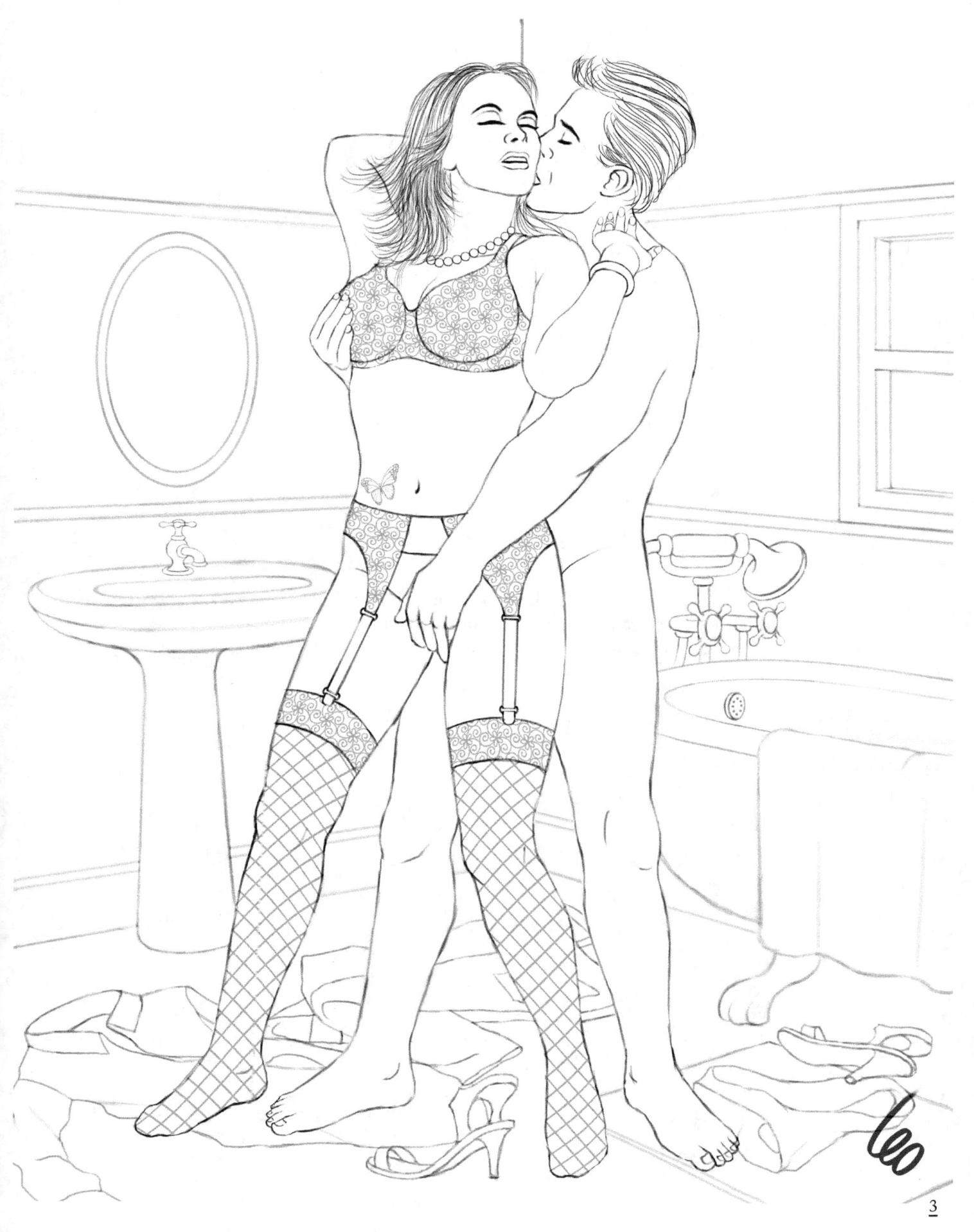

Scene 1

They were getting ready for their hot night out on the town when their eyes locked and they knew they weren't going to make dinner. Just a glimpse of him nude was enough enticement, and while she initiated the sizzling encounter, he is quick to take charge.

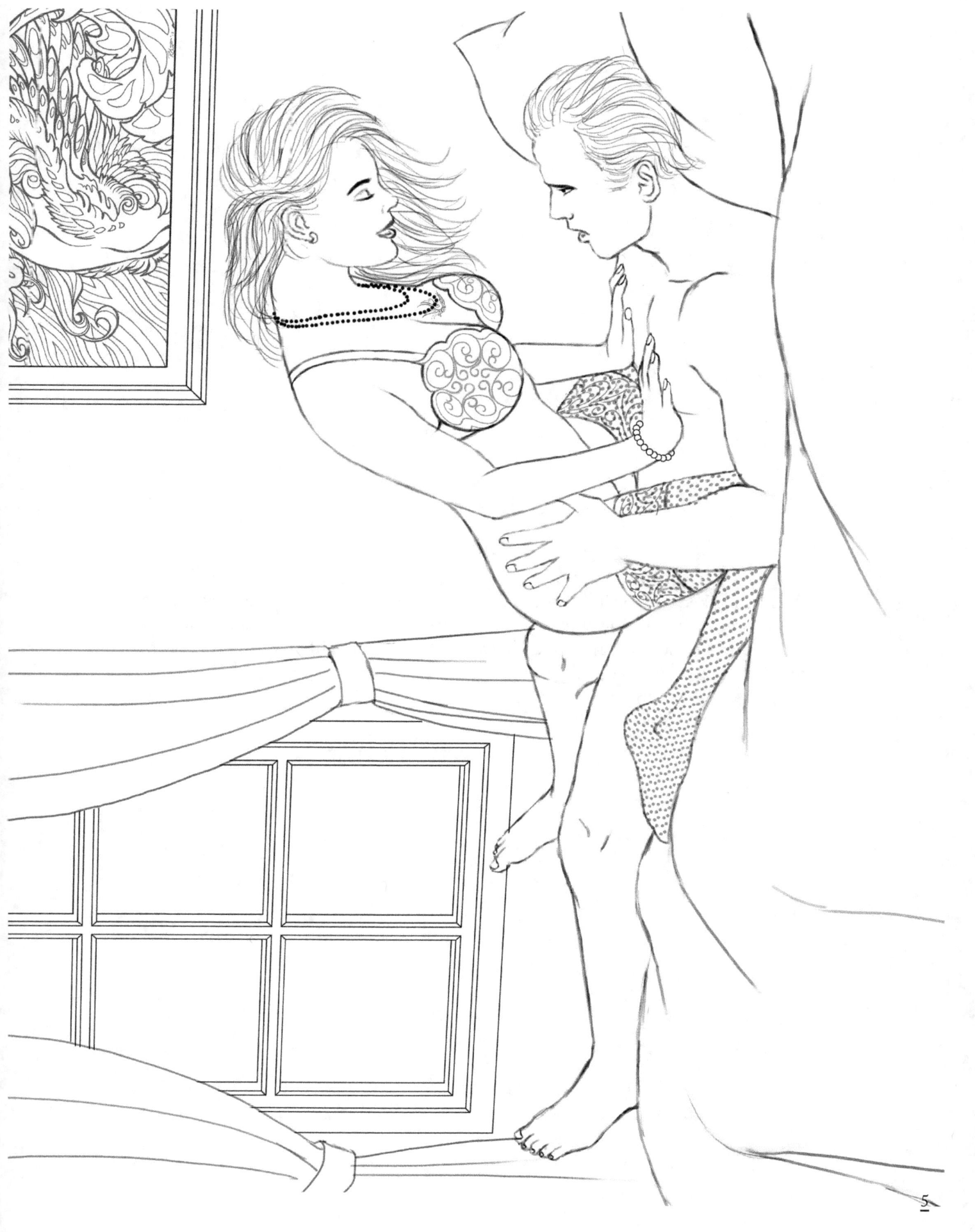

Scene 2

An inviting bed and the incomparably soft afternoon light is the perfect background for amorous love-making and only emphasizes the glow of her skin as she rides her partner. His hands and arms slide between the expanse of her sleek skin and the delicious lace of her thigh-highs.

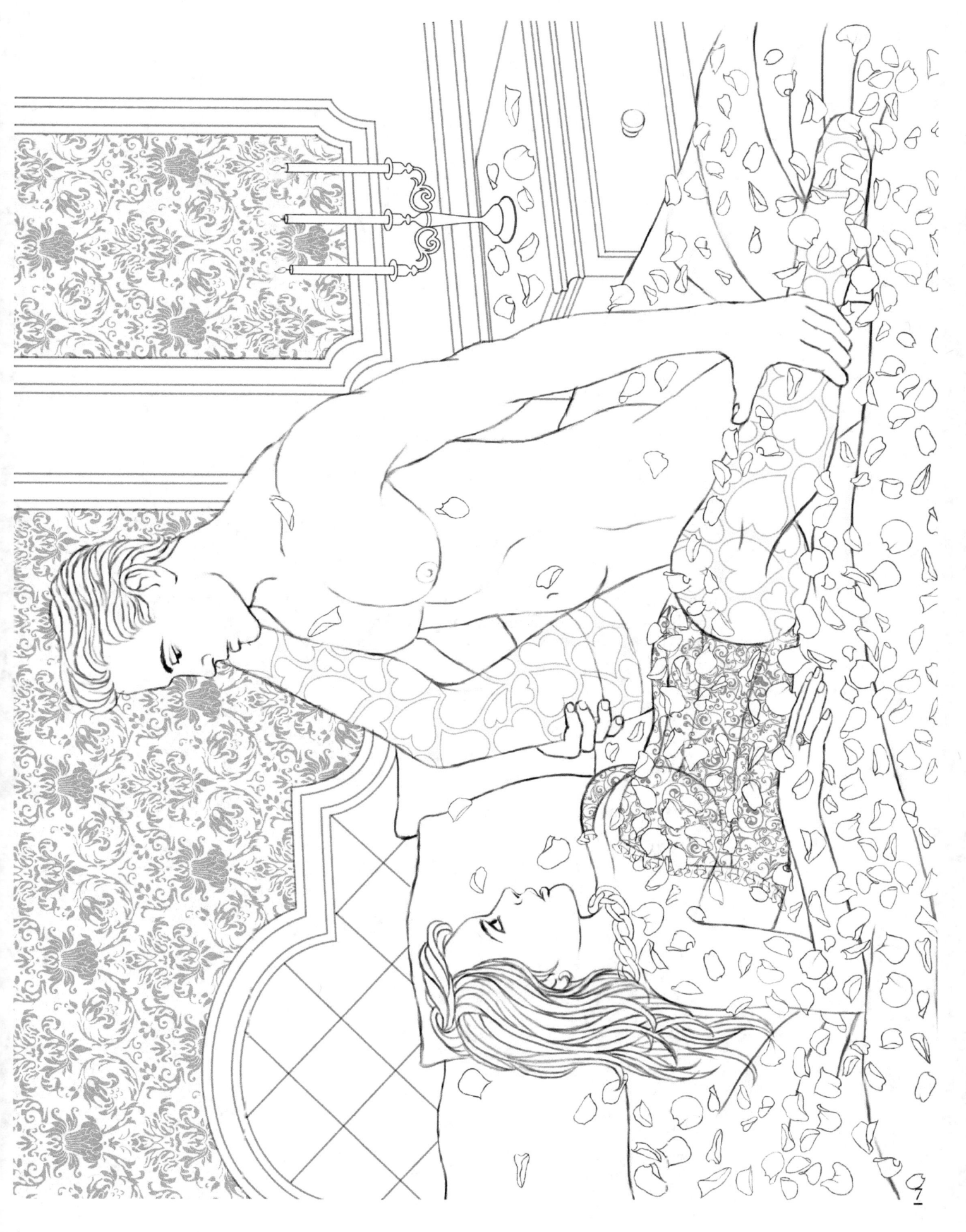

Scene 3

A candlelit boudoir, the intoxicating scent and velvety luxuriousness of rose petals…
and him, in all his strength and intensity. She picked her saucy corset with the intent
of grabbing his attention, and he is showing his appreciation by grabbing her legs in
a delightful display of Gurgent need.

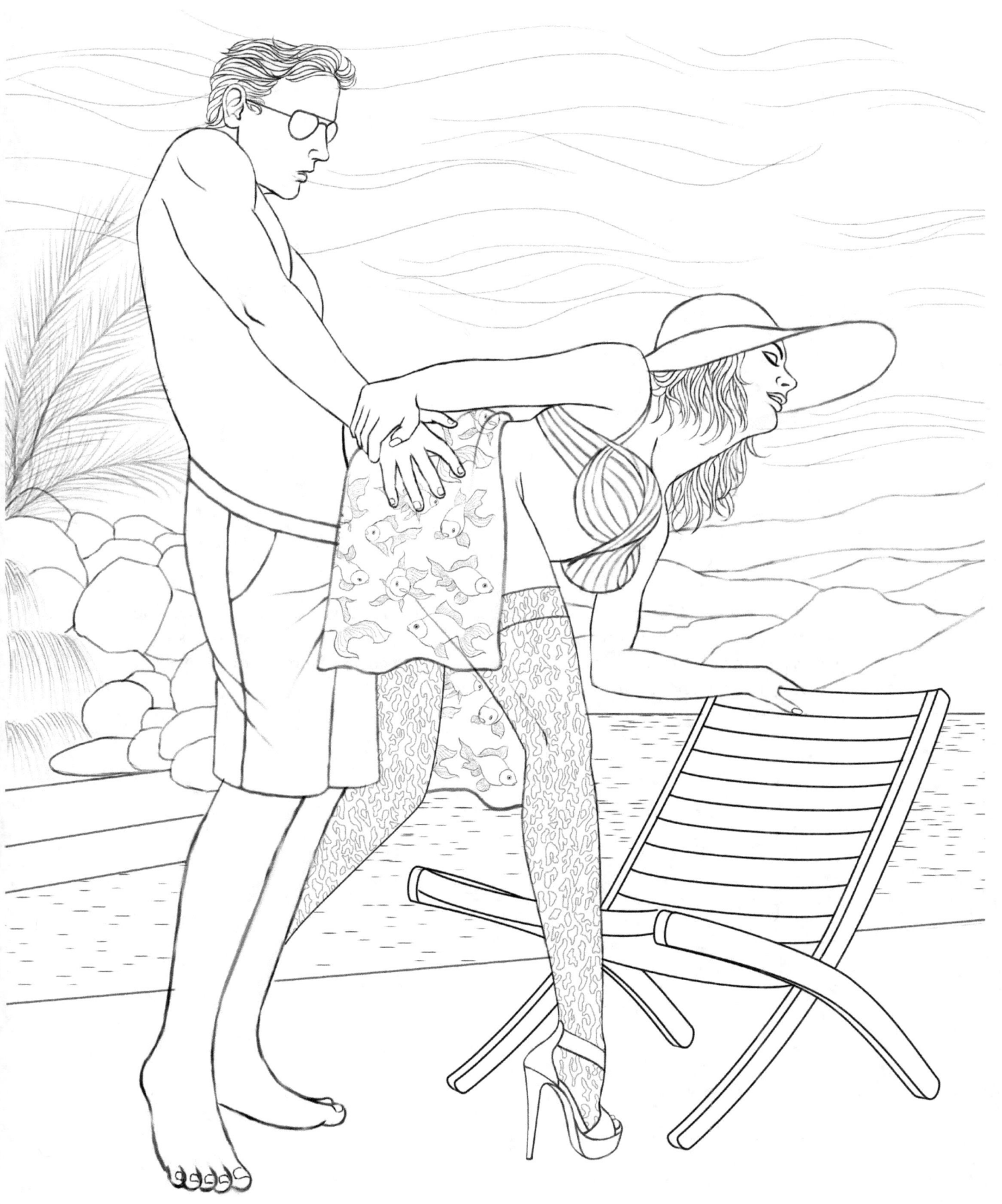

Scene 4

The sybaritic sea air…the tantalizing teases of skin and curves…there is something about vacation that recommends adventurous, naughty play in semi-public spaces where anyone could see. He bends her over the beach chair to show her exactly what he was thinking about while she was tanning.

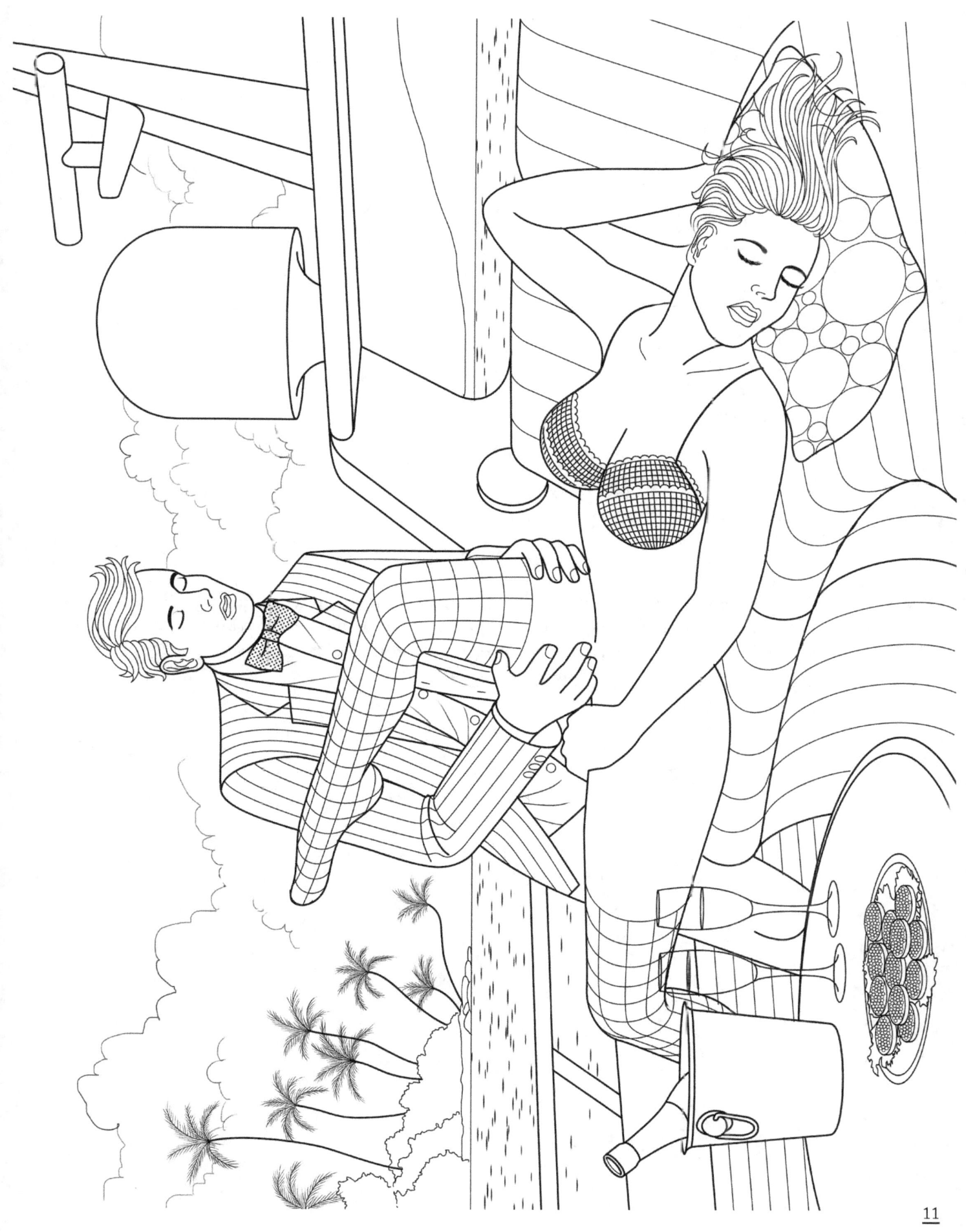

Scene 5

Every once in a while sex should be gloriously decadent, and nothing says "luxe life" like an uninhibited encounter on a private yacht. Who needs bubbly and hors d'oeuvres when you have two ravenous sexual appetites and two lovers who cannot get enough of each other's bodies?

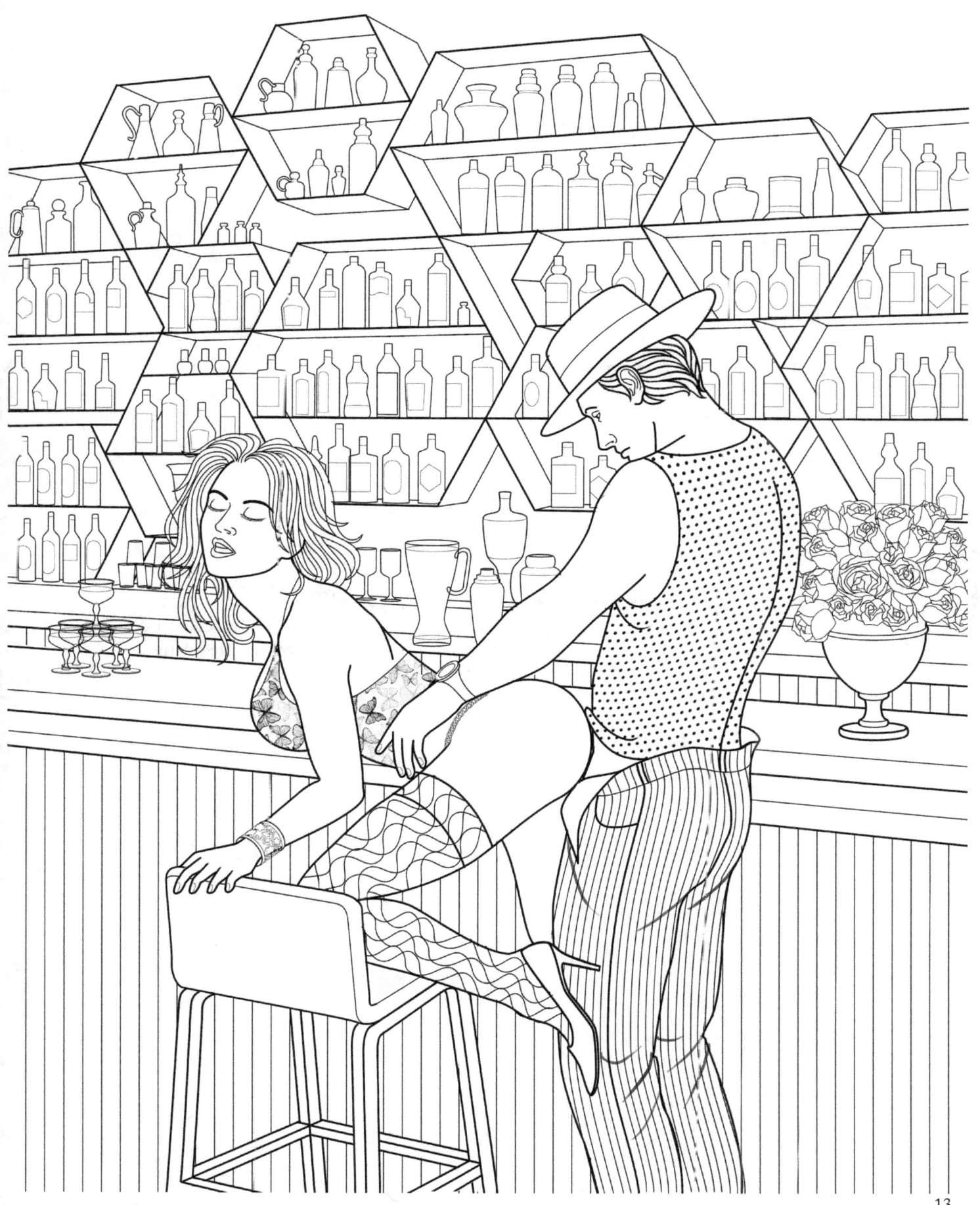

Scene 6

One hot after-hours hook-up — served straight up, please! These lovers don't need any drinks to get right to the point — and get busy. Wine might steal the senses, but in this case the exquisite curve of her rump was the true source of his intoxication.

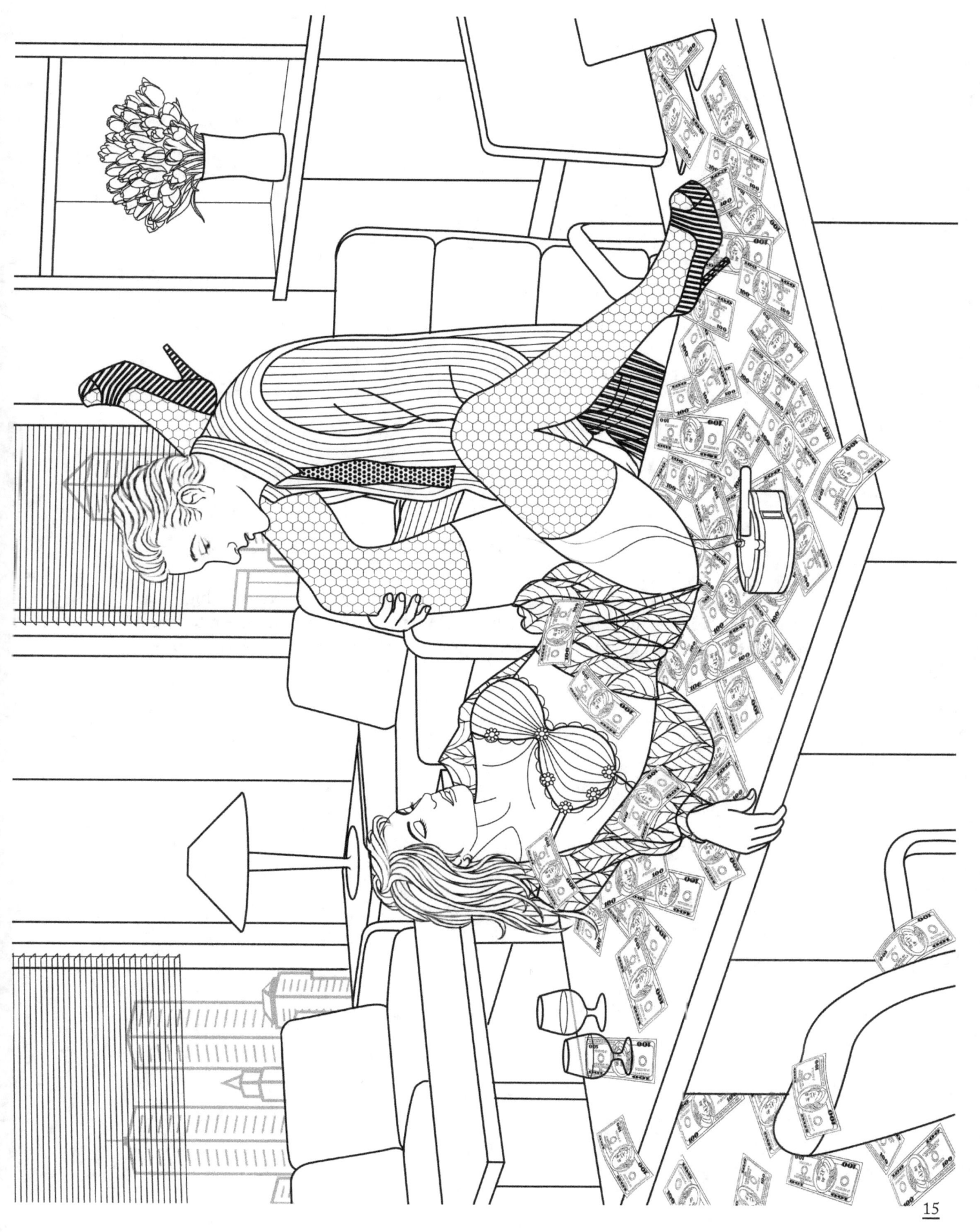

15

Scene 7

The extravagant piles of cash…the incomparable view from a luxurious high-rise penthouse…and her, in fishnets and stilettos. When he tore her shirt open to reveal that alluring lingerie it was "game on" — and in this game, the ante is definitely going up, up, up!

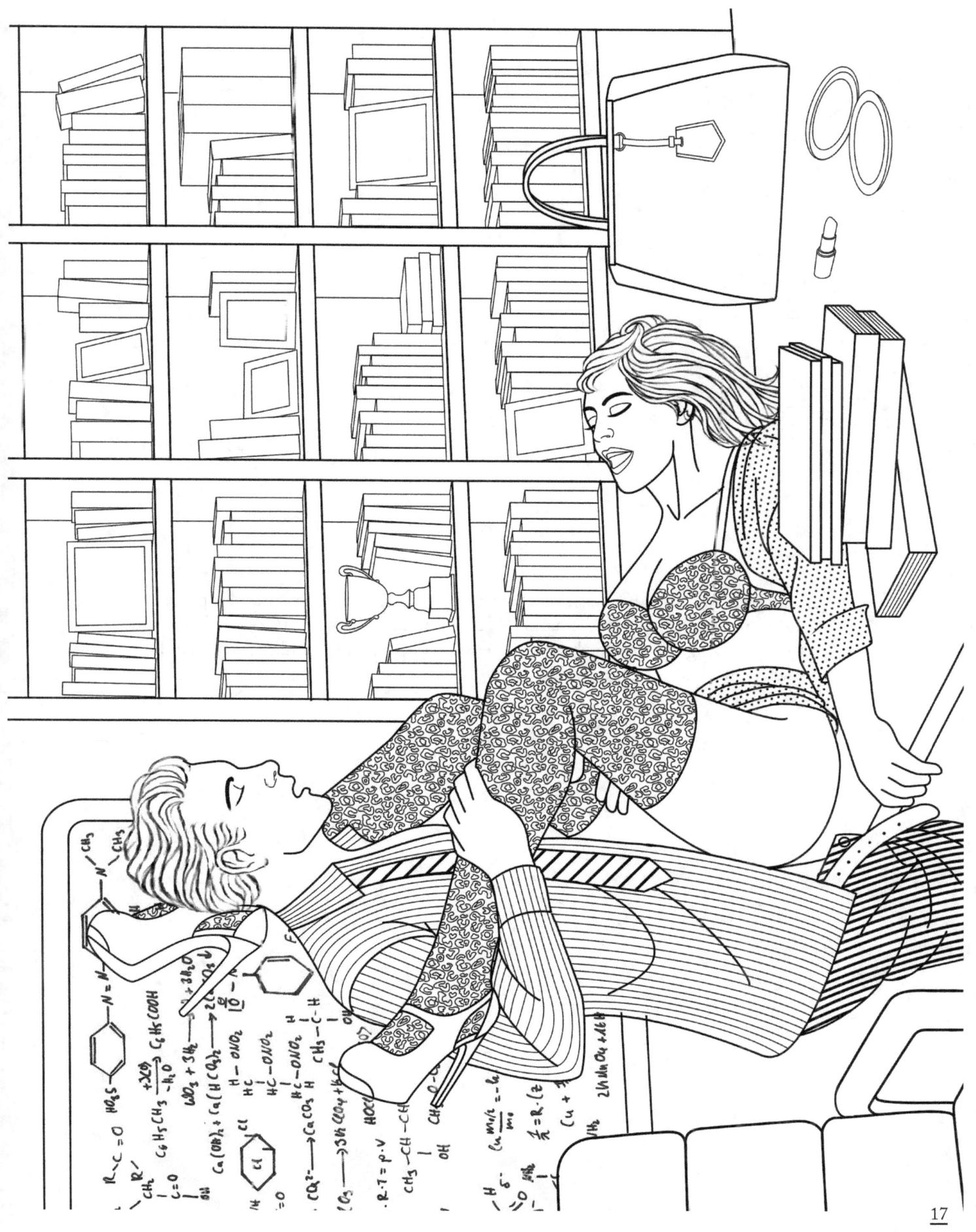

Scene 8

Going back to school has been very rewarding for her, especially since the professor is so willing and able to lend a hand — among other things — after class. Then she started applying lipstick to those full, sensuous lips, and he couldn't resist finding out what she'd do for extra credit.

This page intentionally left blank.

ABOUT THE BOOK

This collection of hot couples illustrations for coloring is sure to heat up any night. Get out your crayons and get in a playful mood. Whether it's at a yacht, the beach, the office or at a sexy nightclub these hot men and women are sure to arouse the sensual side in yourself.